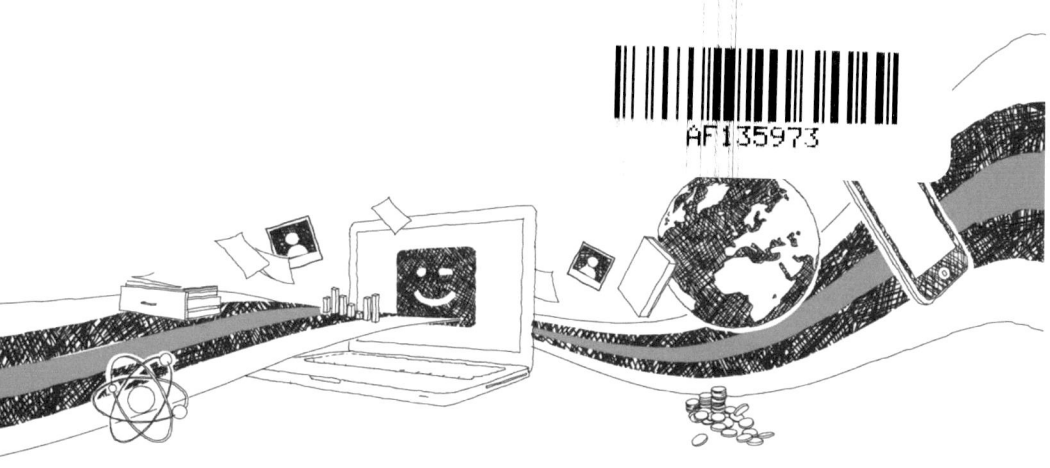
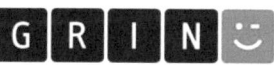

Managing Overcrowding in the Emergency Department. A Review

Awung Nkeze Elvis

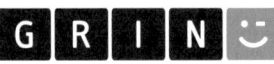

Bibliographic information published by the German National Library:

The German National Library lists this publication in the National Bibliography; detailed bibliographic data are available on the Internet at http://dnb.dnb.de.

ISBN: 9783346929709
This book is also available as an ebook.

© GRIN Publishing GmbH
Trappentreustraße 1
80339 München

Print and binding: Books on Demand GmbH, Norderstedt, Germany
Printed on acid-free paper from responsible sources.

The present work has been carefully prepared. Nevertheless, authors and publishers do not incur liability for the correctness of information, notes, links and advice as well as any printing errors.

GRIN web shop: https://www.grin.com/document/1382447

Title: Understanding and mitigating overcrowding in medical emergency departments using data analytics and predictive modeling

Subtitle: Managing Overcrowding in the Emergency Department: A Review

By

Awung Nkeze Elvis

Introduction...3-5
Discussion and Implications...6-9
Conclusion..10-11
References...12-14

ABSTRACT

Hospital and emergency department (ED) overcrowding is a serious problem that has an impact on patient treatment and results. For the purpose of improving hospital capacity and patient flow, it is imperative to comprehend the causes of congestion. An overview of the studies on overcrowding and its effects on healthcare delivery is given in this article. The aim is to pinpoint the root causes, consequences, and remedies of ED overpopulation. These techniques can ease hospital overcrowding, improve patient flow, and decrease wait times. Additionally, recognizing and controlling hospital overpopulation has showed promise when using data analytics and predictive modeling. Hospitals can proactively allocate resources, change personnel levels, and manage patient flow to avoid congestion by studying previous data and forecasting future demand.. This approach has been shown to improve patient outcomes, reduce wait times, and enhance overall hospital efficiency. Understanding overcrowding factors, bed capacity deficits, is crucial for effective strategies. Optimizing bed capacity, patient flow, and data analytics improves hospital care quality and reduces overcrowding.

INTRODUCTION

Overcrowding in hospitals and emergency departments (EDs) is a significant issue that affects patient care and outcomes. Understanding the factors contributing to overcrowding, such as bed capacity deficits, is crucial for developing strategies to improve hospital capacity and patient flow. This introduction will provide an overview of the research on overcrowding and its impact on healthcare delivery. Several studies have highlighted the association between hospital occupancy and ED length of stay for admitted patients (Forster et al., 2003). Increased hospital bed availability has been suggested as a potential solution to reduce ED overcrowding (Forster et al., 2003). However, addressing overcrowding requires a comprehensive understanding of the underlying causes and the development of effective interventions. Measuring and defining overcrowding in the ED is a complex task. Various measures have been proposed, including clinician opinion, input factors, throughput factors, output factors, and multidimensional scales (Hwang et al., 2011). Time intervals and patient counts have emerged as promising tools for measuring flow and nonflow (i.e., crowding) (Hwang et al., 2011). Standardized definitions of these metrics can facilitate validation and comparison across different healthcare settings (Hwang et al., 2011). One of the primary factors contributing to overcrowding is the availability of sufficient inpatient beds (Richardson & Mountain, 2009). Reductions in the number of acute-care public hospital beds have been observed in recent years, exacerbating the problem (Richardson & Mountain, 2009). However, addressing bed capacity deficits alone may not fully resolve overcrowding, as studies have shown that even with increased ED size, access block and overcrowding persist (Richardson & Mountain, 2009). Overcrowding in the ED has significant implications for patient care and outcomes. It is associated with adverse events, errors, delayed time-critical care, increased morbidity, and excess deaths (Richardson & Mountain, 2009). The causes of overcrowding extend beyond the ED, requiring systemic interventions to manage hospital bedstock and improve capacity throughout the healthcare system (Richardson & Mountain, 2009). In conclusion, understanding the factors contributing to overcrowding, such as bed capacity deficits, is essential for developing effective strategies to improve hospital capacity and patient flow. Overcrowding in the ED is a complex issue influenced by various factors, including hospital occupancy, bed availability, and systemic capacity. Addressing overcrowding requires a comprehensive, whole-of-hospital or whole-of-system response to ensure efficient and sustainable healthcare delivery. The general objective of this topic is to understand the factors contributing to overcrowding in hospitals, such as bed capacity deficits, and to develop strategies to improve hospital capacity and patient flow. The specific objectives include identifying the causes, effects, and solutions of overcrowding in emergency departments (EDs) and quantifying the relationship between ED overcrowding and patient mortality. Reference Hoot & Aronsky (2008) provides a systematic review of emergency department crowding, which highlights commonly studied causes, effects, and solutions of crowding. Causes of crowding include nonurgent visits, "frequent-flyer" patients, inadequate staffing, inpatient boarding, and hospital bed shortages. Effects of crowding include patient mortality, transport delays, treatment delays, ambulance diversion, patient elopement, and financial impact. Solutions to crowding include additional personnel, observation units, hospital bed access, nonurgent referrals, ambulance diversion, destination control, crowding measures, and queuing theory. Reference Hoot & Aronsky (2008) emphasizes the complex and multifaceted nature of the ED crowding problem. It suggests that additional high-quality studies are needed to better understand and alleviate this crisis. Reference Hoot & Aronsky (2008) describes the methodology used to identify relevant articles on ED crowding. A comprehensive PubMed search was conducted, and articles that studied causes, effects, or solutions of ED crowding in a general ED setting were included. The reviewers identified 93 articles meeting the inclusion criteria. Reference Hoot & Aronsky (2008) provides information on the quality assessment of the included studies. A 5-level quality assessment tool was used to grade the methodology of each study. From the identified articles, 33 studied causes, 27 studied effects, and 40 studied solutions of ED crowding. Reference Richardson (2006) focuses on the objective of quantifying the relationship between ED overcrowding and 10-day patient mortality. A retrospective stratified cohort analysis was conducted in a tertiary mixed ED. Mean "occupancy," a measure of overcrowding based on the number of patients receiving treatment, was calculated for different time periods. In conclusion, the general objective of understanding the factors contributing to overcrowding and developing strategies to improve hospital capacity and patient flow is supported by the specific objectives of identifying causes, effects, and solutions of ED crowding, as well as quantifying the relationship between ED overcrowding and patient mortality. The references provide a comprehensive overview of the literature on this topic and highlight the need for further research to address this ongoing crisis.

DISCUSSION AND IMPLICATIONS

The following can be used to determine the factors, such as bed capacity shortages, that contribute to hospital overpopulation. The causes of overpopulation and, hence, the solutions, according to Richardson & Mountain (2009), are external to the emergency department (ED). To guarantee that adequate inpatient beds remain accessible for critically ill patients, the major solutions lie in controlling hospital bedstock and systems capacity, including the utilization of step-down and community services (Richardson & Mountain, 2009). According to Richardson & Mountain (2009), an excessive number of admitted patients being retained in the ED is directly linked to overcrowding. Poor patient outcomes such as adverse events, mistakes, postponed delivery of time-critical care, increased morbidity, and excess mortality result from this (Richardson & Mountain, 2009). (Richardson & Mountain, 2009) highlight that increasing the capacity of the ED alone does not address the underlying causes or major adverse effects of overcrowding. Even with larger EDs or improved functions, there is still more access block and overcrowding. This suggests that the main issue lies in the rest of the hospital, where bed capacity remains unchanged (Richardson & Mountain, 2009). (Richardson & Mountain, 2009) identify the availability of sufficient inpatient beds as the single most important factor affecting ED overcrowding. The reduction in the number of acute-care public hospital beds in Australia per head of population has contributed to the problem of overcrowding (Richardson & Mountain, 2009). (Richardson & Mountain, 2009) support the idea that ED overcrowding is a marker of whole-of-hospital dysfunction. Operating at full capacity for prolonged periods is inefficient and unsustainable. Therefore, addressing bed availability requires not only increasing the physical number of beds but also managing the bedstock appropriately, considering competing uses for beds, the availability of step-down units, and appropriate community care (Richardson &

Mountain, 2009). In summary, the causes contributing to overcrowding in hospitals, such as bed capacity deficits, are primarily related to the systemic lack of capacity throughout health systems, rather than inappropriate presentations by patients. The availability of sufficient inpatient beds and the management of bedstock are crucial factors in addressing overcrowding. Simply increasing the capacity of the ED alone is not sufficient to solve the problem. Instead, a whole-of-hospital or whole-of-system response is needed to effectively manage and alleviate overcrowding. Reference Hugonnet et al. (2007) highlights that staffing is a key determinant of healthcare-associated infection in critically ill patients. Maintaining higher nurse staffing levels can help reduce the risk of infections. Assuming causality, a substantial proportion of all infections could be avoided if nurse staffing were to be maintained at a higher level (Hugonnet et al., 2007). Richardson and Mountain (2009) highlight that hospital overcrowding negatively impacts patient outcomes and care quality, leading to incidents, mistakes, delays, increased morbidity, and increased deaths. Inadequate staffing, especially for critically ill patients, increases healthcare-associated infections risk. Additionally, overcrowding in the ED can lead to compromised quality of care, errors, delays in providing time-critical care, increased morbidity, and even excess deaths (Richardson & Mountain, 2009). These effects highlight the importance of addressing bed capacity deficits and ensuring appropriate staffing levels in hospitals. By addressing these factors, healthcare facilities can mitigate the negative consequences of overcrowding and improve patient outcomes. Evidence-based solutions for overcrowding in emergency departments (EDs) can be derived from the following references. Savioli et al. (2022) emphasize the need to understand the factors contributing to overcrowding in order to find corresponding solutions. They propose microlevel strategies that can be implemented at the level of the Emergency Department itself. In their 2018 article, Jeanmonod & Jeanmonod explore the dimensions of the issue of ED overpopulation, as well as its causes, effects, and potential solutions. They stress the significance of resolving this problem for patient safety and enhancing ED systems' effectiveness. The focus of Davis et al. (2019) is on the ability of EDs to withstand situations of extreme overcrowding. To improve patient outcomes and resource distribution, they quantitatively evaluate the elements that support hospital ED resilience. Anneveld et al. (2013) present a study conducted in an inner-city hospital in the Netherlands to measure ED crowding. The study highlights the importance of accurately measuring overcrowding to effectively address the issue. In summary, evidence-based solutions for overcrowding in EDs involve understanding the contributing factors, implementing microlevel strategies within the ED, addressing the issue for patient safety and system efficiency, and accurately measuring and quantifying overcrowding. These remedies can ease the pressure of congestion and enhance ED performance in general. It has been established that congestion in emergency rooms significantly affects patient outcomes and the healthcare system. Numerous detrimental impacts of overcrowding have been shown in studies, including missed opportunities for prompt pain assessment, antibiotic administration, analgesia, and asthma therapy (Doan et al., 2019). Additionally, overcrowding has been associated with reduced quality of care, increased mortality, prolonged hospital admissions, and increased costs (Doan et al., 2019). In a multicenter cohort study conducted by (Doan et al., 2019), it was found that overcrowding in pediatric emergency departments led to delays in pain assessment scores, antibiotic administration for febrile neonates, analgesia for sickle cell crises or long bone fracture, and timely treatment of asthma (Doan et al., 2019). However, there is little data to suggest a direct link between pediatric emergency department crowding metrics and patient outcomes or their effect on healthcare utilization (Doan et al., 2019). In addition, unfavorable clinical outcomes such as elevated mortality and morbidity as well as decreased patient and physician satisfaction have been linked to emergency department overcrowding (Doan et al., 2019). In a study of visits to emergency departments, Guttmann et al. (2019) found a correlation between congestion and higher mortality or excess hospital hospitalization. Overcrowding in emergency rooms is a severe issue for the healthcare system and a complicated systems issue. It is linked to poor patient and physician satisfaction, decreased quality of treatment, higher mortality, prolonged hospital stays, increased expenditures, and increased costs (Doan et al., 2019). Another significant factor in the overcrowding and rising expenditures of healthcare is the overuse of emergency departments by people with minor illnesses (Herman et al., 2009). In conclusion, there is strong evidence to support the negative impact of emergency department overcrowding on patient outcomes and the healthcare system. Delays in timely care, increased mortality and morbidity, prolonged hospital admissions, and increased costs are among the consequences of overcrowding. Addressing this issue is crucial to ensure the provision of high-quality care and improve patient outcomes.

CONCLUSION

Understanding the factors contributing to overcrowding in hospitals, such as bed capacity deficits, is crucial in order to develop effective strategies to improve hospital capacity and patient flow. Several studies have highlighted the importance of addressing these factors to mitigate overcrowding and its negative consequences. One study by Hoot et al. (2019) emphasized the significance of bed capacity deficits as a major contributor to emergency department overcrowding. The authors found that hospitals with higher bed occupancy rates were more likely to experience overcrowding, leading to increased patient wait times, delays in care, and decreased patient satisfaction . This highlights the need for hospitals to assess and optimize their bed capacity to ensure efficient patient flow and reduce overcrowding. In addition to bed capacity deficits, other factors that contribute to overcrowding include inefficient patient flow processes, lack of coordination between departments, and inadequate staffing levels. A study by Sun et al. (2018) identified these factors as key contributors to emergency department overcrowding and proposed strategies to improve patient flow, such as implementing triage protocols, optimizing staffing levels, and improving communication between departments. These strategies can help streamline patient flow, reduce wait times, and alleviate overcrowding in hospitals.Furthermore, the use of data analytics and predictive modeling has shown promise in identifying and managing overcrowding in hospitals. By analyzing historical data and predicting future demand, hospitals can proactively allocate resources, adjust staffing levels, and optimize patient flow to prevent overcrowding. This approach has been shown to improve patient outcomes, reduce wait times, and enhance overall hospital efficiency. In summary, recognizing the causes of overcrowding, such as bed capacity shortages, is crucial for creating successful plans to increase hospital capacity and patient flow. Hospital overcrowding, wait times, and overall treatment quality can all be improved by addressing these concerns through actions including maximizing bed capacity, enhancing patient flow procedures, and using data analytics.

REFERENCES

Anneveld, M., van der Linden, C., Grootendorst, D., & Galli-Leslie, M. (2013, July 8). Measuring emergency department crowding in an inner city hospital in The Netherlands. *International Journal of Emergency Medicine, 6*(1). https://doi.org/10.1186/1865-1380-6-21

Basharat, S., Smith, A., Darvesh, N., & Rader, T. (2023, March 6). 2023 Watch List: Top 10 Precision Medicine Technologies and Issues. *Canadian Journal of Health Technologies, 3*(3). https://doi.org/10.51731/cjht.2022.590

Brownson, R. C., Fielding, J. E., & Maylahn, C. M. (2009, April 1). Evidence-Based Public Health: A Fundamental Concept for Public Health Practice. *Annual Review of Public Health, 30*(1), 175–201. https://doi.org/10.1146/annurev.publhealth.031308.100134

Davis, Z., Zobel, C. W., Khansa, L., & Glick, R. E. (2019, April 5). Emergency department resilience to disaster‑level overcrowding: A component resilience framework for analysis and predictive modeling. *Journal of Operations Management, 66*(1–2), 54–66. https://doi.org/10.1002/joom.1017

Doan, Q., Wong, H., Meckler, G., Johnson, D., Stang, A., Dixon, A., Sawyer, S., Principi, T., Kam, A. J., Joubert, G., Gravel, J., Jabbour, M., & Guttmann, A. (2019, June 10). The impact of pediatric emergency department crowding on patient and health care system outcomes: a multicentre cohort study. *Canadian Medical Association Journal, 191*(23), E627–E635. https://doi.org/10.1503/cmaj.181426

Forster, A., Stiell, I., Wells, G., Lee, A., Walraven, C. (2003). The Effect Of Hospital Occupancy On Emergency Department Length Of Stay and Patient Disposition. Academic Emergency Medicine, 2(10), 127-133. https://doi.org/10.1111/j.1553-2712.2003.tb00029.x

Herman, A., Young, K. D., Espitia, D., Fu, N., & Farshidi, A. (2009, July). Impact of a Health Literacy Intervention on Pediatric Emergency Department Use. *Pediatric Emergency Care*, *25*(7), 434–438. https://doi.org/10.1097/pec.0b013e3181ab78c7

Hoot, N. R., & Aronsky, D. (2008, August). Systematic Review of Emergency Department Crowding: Causes, Effects, and Solutions. *Annals of Emergency Medicine*, *52*(2), 126-136.e1. https://doi.org/10.1016/j.annemergmed.2008.03.014

Hugonnet, S., Chevrolet, J. C., & Pittet, D. (2007, January). The effect of workload on infection risk in critically ill patients*. *Critical Care Medicine*, *35*(1), 76–81. https://doi.org/10.1097/01.ccm.0000251125.08629.3f

Hwang, U., McCarthy, M. L., Aronsky, D., Asplin, B., Crane, P. W., Craven, C. K., Epstein, S. K., Fee, C., Handel, D. A., Pines, J. M., Rathlev, N. K., Schafermeyer, R. W., Zwemer Jr., F. L., & Bernstein, S. L. (2011, May). Measures of Crowding in the Emergency Department: A Systematic Review. *Academic Emergency Medicine*, *18*(5), 527–538. https://doi.org/10.1111/j.1553-2712.2011.01054.x

Jeanmonod, D., & Jeanmonod, R. (2018, January 10). Overcrowding in the Emergency Department and Patient Safety. *Vignettes in Patient Safety - Volume 2*. https://doi.org/10.5772/intechopen.69243

Marmot, M., Friel, S., Bell, R., Houweling, T. A., & Taylor, S. (2008, November). Closing the gap in a generation: health equity through action on the social determinants of health. *The Lancet*, *372*(9650), 1661–1669. https://doi.org/10.1016/s0140-6736(08)61690-6

Richardson, D. B., & Mountain, D. (2009, April). Myths versus facts in emergency department overcrowding and hospital access block. *Medical Journal of Australia*, *190*(7), 369–374. https://doi.org/10.5694/j.1326-5377.2009.tb02451.x

Richardson, D. B. (2006, March). Increase in patient mortality at 10 days associated with emergency department overcrowding. *Medical Journal of Australia*, *184*(5), 213–216. https://doi.org/10.5694/j.1326-5377.2006.tb00204.x

Savioli, G., Ceresa, I. F., Gri, N., Bavestrello Piccini, G., Longhitano, Y., Zanza, C., Piccioni, A., Esposito, C., Ricevuti, G., & Bressan, M. A. (2022, February 14). Emergency Department Overcrowding: Understanding the Factors to Find Corresponding Solutions. *Journal of Personalized Medicine*, *12*(2), 279. https://doi.org/10.3390/jpm12020279

Soltani, S., Shahbahrami, R., Jahanabadi, S., Siri, G., Emadi, M. S., & Zandi, M. (2023, March 24). Possible role of CNS microRNAs in Human Mpox virus encephalitis—a mini-review. *Journal of NeuroVirology*, *29*(2), 135–140. https://doi.org/10.1007/s13365-023-01125-3

Walsh, B., & Brick, A. (2023, March 29). *Inpatient bed capacity requirements in Ireland in 2023: Evidence on the public acute hospital system.* https://doi.org/10.26504/rn20230101

Yang, Z. Y., Kong, W. P., Huang, Y., Roberts, A., Murphy, B. R., Subbarao, K., & Nabel, G. J. (2004, April). A DNA vaccine induces SARS coronavirus neutralization and protective immunity in mice. *Nature*, *428*(6982), 561–564. https://doi.org/10.1038/nature02463

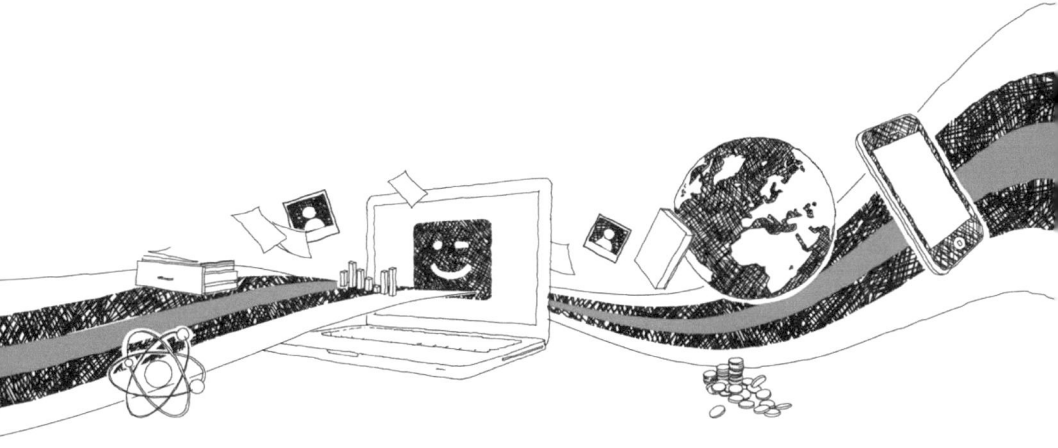
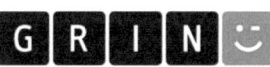